150 Anywhere Workouts:

High Intensity Bodyweight Training Anytime

By: Fred Hughes

I am dedicated to serving the public and helping others achieve their physical or mental goals. I believe that fitness is one of the core components for living a successful life. I have spent the last 10 years formulating and testing fitness regiments. With 5 years in the United States Marine Corps Infantry, 2 years of Diplomatic Security, 4 total deployments to austere locations, and certifications in both Personal Training and High Intensity Training, my programs are proven to increase athletic performance.

This program is a **master list** of **150 No Equipment** workout routines created over the past 10 years. The routines are hard but they work. Stick with the program and complete as many reps/rounds as possible. Keep fighting and push the body above self-imposed limitations to achieve a higher level of performance.

*Scale to individual athletic performance if unable to complete total workout.

Recommended Split:
4 Days On
1 Day Off
Program's 4 on 1 off Split:
Upper Body
Lower Body
Cardio/Abs
Full Body
Active Rest/Recovery

Anywhere - Anytime - Always Ready

All the workouts in this book require no gym and can be completed at home or on the road. The average completion time per workout is 30 minutes or less.

Example of 1 Body Weight Workout Routine:

3 Rounds for Time:
10 Burpees
20 1 and ¼ Air Squats
20 Jumping Lunges (10 Each Leg)
30 Mountain Climbers
50 Standing Elbow to Knee Crunches
Time: _____

Example of 1 Cardio and Ab Workout Routine:

10 - 50 Meter Sprints (30 Seconds Rest Between Each)
100 Flutter Kicks
100 Russian Twists
100 Jumping Jacks
100 High Knees (Running in Place)
Time: _____

Waiver of Liability

Workout 1:
3 Rounds for Time:

25 1 and ¼ Squats
25 Long Jump with Backward Jog to Start
25 High Knees
25 Flutter Kicks
25 Standing Calf Raise
24 Jumping Lunges (12 Per Leg)
25 Bicycle Crunches
Time: _____

Workout 2:
For Time:

10 X 100 Meter Sprints (No more than 30 Seconds
Between Sprints)
Then:
100 Standing Knee to Elbow
100 Jumping Jacks
Time: _____

Workout 3:
5 Rounds for Time:

50 Seconds of Shadow Boxing
50 Mountain Climbers
50 Jumping Jacks
50 High Knees
50 Flutter Kicks
Time: _____

Workout 4:

Max Repetitions (1 Minute Break Between Workouts):

2 Minutes of Flutter Kicks
2 Minutes of Jumping Jacks
2 Minutes of Push Ups
2 Minutes of Sit Ups
2 Minutes of Mountain Climbers
Reps: ____ ____ ____ ____ ____

Workout 5:
As Many Rounds as Possible in 15 Minutes:

20 Lunges (10 Each Leg)
20 Bench Dips
20 Air Squats
20 Crunches/Sit Ups
Rounds Completed: _____

Workout 6:
5 Rounds for Time:

10 Incline Push Ups
10 Sit Ups
10 Decline Push Ups
10 Sit Ups
10 Push Ups
10 Sit Ups
100 Jumping Jacks
Time: _____

Workout 7:
For Time:

1 Mile Run
100 Flutter Kicks
20 Long Jumps with Backward Jog to Start Point
20 Meter Sprint
100 Russian Twists
20 Meter Backward Sprint
Time: _____

Workout 8:
3 Rounds for Time:

20 Jumping Lunges
20 Burpees
20 V-Ups
10 Dive Bomber Push Ups
20 Squat Jumps
20 Jumping Jacks
20 Plank Walkouts (Hand Walkout)
Time: _____

Workout 9:
3 Rounds for Time:

20 Meter Crab Walk
20 Close Grip Push Ups
20 Bench Dips
20 Meter Bear Crawl
20 Incline Push Ups
Time: _____

<u>Workout 10</u>:
3 Rounds for Time:

20 Air Squats
20 Push-Ups
30 Standing Knee to Elbow
40 Calf Raises
50 Jumping Jacks
Time: _____

<u>Workout 11</u>:
3 Rounds for Time:

50 Mountain Climbers
50 Reverse Crunches
50 High Knees
30 Flutter Kicks
30 Jumping Jacks
30 Alternating Toe Taps
Time: _____

<u>Workout 12</u>:
3 Rounds for Time:

20 Incline Push Ups
20 Plank Crunches
50 Side Large Arm Circles Forward
50 Side Large Arm Circles Backwards
50 Flutter Kicks
50 Jumping Jacks
Time: _____

Workout 13:
5 Rounds for Time:

20 Air Squats
200 Meters Run
20 Push Ups
20 High Knees
Time: _____

Workout 14:
For Time:

1-Mile Jog (Throughout Jog Sprint 10 Seconds at Least
10 Times)
100 Jumping Jacks
50 Flutter Kicks
Time: _____

Workout 15:
3 Rounds for Time:

15 Burpees
20 Push Ups
25 Bench/Chair Dips
30 Flutter Kicks
35 Mountain Climbers
40 Sit Ups
50 Alternating Toe Taps
Time: _____

Workout 16:
3 Rounds for Time:

10 8-Count Push Ups
20 Burpees with Push Ups
30 Standing Knee to Elbow
40 Russian Twists
50 Jumping Jacks
Time: _____

Workout 17:
3 Rounds for Time:

30 Second Bridge Pose
30 Second Left Side Plank
30 Second Plank Crunches
30 Second Right Side Plank
30 Large Arm Circles Forward
30 Large Arm Circles Backward
30 Overhead Air Press
30 V-Ups
Time: _____

Workout 18:
3 Rounds of Time:

10 Pistol Squats (Per Leg)
20 Jumping Lunges
30 Mountain Climbers
40 Straight Leg Toe Touches
50 Standing Knee to Elbow
Time: _____

Workout 19:
For Time:

Run/Jog 1 Mile
20 Push Ups
20 Meter Bear Crawl
40 Flutter Kicks
50 Russian Twists
50 Jumping Jacks
Time: _____

Workout 20:
3 Rounds for Time:

40 Jumping Squats
25 Left Side Crunches
25 Right Side Crunches
40 Standing Calf Raises
40 Lunges
Time: _____

Workout 21:
10 Rounds for Time:

10 Push Ups
20 Crunches
10 Bench Dips
20 Alternating Toe Taps
Time: _____

Workout 22:
For Time:

99 Flutter Kicks
99 Jumping Jacks
99 Mountain Climbers
99 Core Twists with Feet Lifted
99 Bunny Hops
100 High Knees
Time: _____

Workout 23:
For Time:

100 Push Ups
100 Air Squats
100 Flutter Kicks
100 Bench Dips
100 Russian Twists
25 Burpees
Time: _____

Workout 24:
3 Rounds for Time:

20 Mountain Climbers
20 Alt Toe Taps
20 Second Wall Walk
20 Second Star Plank
20 Second Bridge Pose
20 Meter Crab Walk
Time: _____

Workout 25:
3 Rounds for Time:

50 Jumping Jacks
5 Burpees
50 High Knees
5 Burpees
50 Crunches
Time: _____

Workout 26:
3 Rounds for Time:

20 Incline Push Ups
20 Reverse Flutter Kicks
20 ¼ Down Handstand Push Ups
20 Jumping Lunges (10 Each Leg)
20 Close Grip Push Ups
20 Ab Wipers
20 Side-to-Side Hop (Feet Together)
Time: _____

Workout 27:
3 Rounds for Time:

25 Bench Dips
25 Push Ups
25 Small Arm Circles Backwards
25 Small Arm Circles Forward
25 OH Air Press
25 Vertical Leg Crunches
Time: _____

Workout 28:
5 Rounds for Time:

15 Mountain Climbers
15 Incline Push Ups
15 Bench Dips
15 Burpees
Time: _____

Workout 29:
For Time:

Jog/Run 1 Mile
50 Air Squats
Jog/Run 1 Mile
50 Walking Lunges
50 Flutter Kicks
Time: _____

Workout 30:
3 Rounds for Time:

50 Standing Knees-to-Elbows Cross
50 Jumping Jacks
50 Flutter Kicks
50 Side-to-Side Hops
50 Mountain Climbers
50 Alt. Toe Taps
Time: _____

Workout 31:
3 Rounds for Time:

30 Sitting Punches (Feet Elevated)
30 Jumping Jacks
30 Second L-Sit
30 Crunches
30 High Knees
30 Ab Wipers
30 Reverse Crunches
Time:_____

Workout 32:
3 Rounds for Time:

10 Burpees
20 Standing Knee to Elbow Crunch
30 Second Star Plank
40 Jumping Jacks
50 Bunny Hops
Time: _____

Workout 33:
4 Rounds for Time:

20 Incline Push Ups
20 Mountain Climbers
20 Decline Push Ups
20 Bicycle Crunches
20 8-Count Push Ups
20 Flutter Kicks
Time: _____

Workout 34:
3 Rounds for Time:

50 Bunny Hops
50 Speed Skaters
50 Jumping Jacks
50 Core Twists with Feet Lifted
50 High Knees
50 Plank Crunches
Time: _____

Workout 35:
3 Rounds for Time:

30 Seconds Wall Sit (Legs 90 degrees back against wall)
30 Second Plank
30 Second Left Side Plank
30 Second Right Side Plank
30 Squat to Calf Raises
Time: _____

Workout 36:
3 Rounds for Time:

20 Burpees
20 Push Ups
50 Bunny Hops
20 Bench Dips
50 Jumping Jacks
20 Decline Push Ups
Time: _____

Workout 37:
For Time:

100 Burpees
100 Bicycle Crunches
100 Alt Toe Taps
100 Jumping Jacks
100 High Knees
Time: _____

Workout 38:
3 Rounds for Time:

20 Jump Squats
40 Bunny Hops
20 Jumping Lunges
40 High Knees
20 Standing Knee to Elbow
40 Mountain Climbers
Time: _____

Workout 39:
3 Rounds for Time:

30 Incline Push Ups
30 V-Ups
30 Overhead Air Press
30 Side Large Arm Circles Forward
30 Side Large Arm Circles Backwards
30 Jumping Jacks
Time: _____

Workout 40:
3 Rounds for Time:

10 Crossover Push Ups (Use Book/Box/Small Platform)
10 Wall Walks (Wall Walkout)
10 Hand Walkouts
10 Burpees with Push Up
10 Body Weight Floor Scorpions
Time: _____

Workout 42:
3 Rounds for Time:

30 Split Squats (15 Each Leg)
30 Standing Straight Leg Toe Touch
30 Bunny Hops
30 Side Lunges (15 Per Side)
30 High Knees
30 Donkey Kicks (15 Per Side)
Time: _____

Workout 43:
3 Rounds for Time:

10 Burpees
15 Jump Squats
20 Lunges (10 Each Leg)
25 Mountain Climbers
30 Flutter Kicks
35 Russian Twists
Time: _____

Workout 44:
3 Rounds for Time:

50 High Knees
50 Bunny Hops
50 Side-to-Side Hops
50 Standing Knee to Elbows
50 Flutter Kicks
Time: _____

Workout 45:
3 Rounds for Time:

20 Incline Push Ups
20 Flutter Kicks
20 Decline Push Ups
20 V-Ups with Twist
20 Close Grip Push Ups
20 Plank Crunches
Time: _____

Workout 46:
3 Rounds for Time:

20 Air Squats
20 Jumping Lunges
20 Bunny Hops
20 Mountain Climbers
20 High Knees
Time: _____

Workout 47:
3 Rounds for Time:

25 Diamond Push Ups
25 Meter Supine Crab Walk
25 Second Star Plank
25 Burpees
25 Incline Push Ups
25 Meter Bear Crawl
25 V-Ups
Time: _____

Workout 48:
3 Rounds for Time:

10 Pistol Squats (Per Leg)
10 Split Squats (Per Leg)
1 Minute Second Wall Sit
1 Minute of Speed Skaters
100 Jumping Jacks
100 Bunny Hops
Time: _____

Workout 49:
For Time:

100 Jumping Jacks
100 High Crunches
100 Mountain Climbers
100 Bicycle Crunches
1 Mile Run/Jog
Time: _____

Workout 50:
5 Rounds for Time:

25 Tuck Jumps
200 Meters Sprint
30 Walking Lunges
35 Plank Crunches
Time: _____

Workout 51:
For Time:

100 Meters of Straight Leg Bound Drill
1-Mile Run
100 Meters of High Skipping Running Drill
Time: _____

Workout 52:
3 Rounds for Time:

50 High Knees
50 Russian Twists
50 Standing Knee-To-Elbow Crunch
50 Jumping Jacks
50 Flutter Kicks
50 High Crunches
Time: _____

Workout 53:
10 Rounds for Time:

10-Meter Skipping Running Drill (High Skip)
100-Meter Sprint
10-Meter Crossover Running Drill Left
10-Meter Crossover Running Drill Right
Time: _____

Workout 54:
3 Rounds for Time:

20 Russian Twists
20 Diamond Push Ups
20 Side Large Forward Arm Circles
20 Side Large Backwards Arm Circles
20 Bench Dips
20 Incline Push Ups
20 V-Ups
Time: _____

Workout 55:
5 Rounds for Time:

20 1 and ¼ Air Squats
20 Jumping Lunges
40 Mountain Climbers
40 V-Ups
40 High Knees
Time: _____

Workout 56:
5 Rounds for Time:

100-Meter Sprint
10 Squat to Long Jump
10 Walking Lunges
10 Burpees
Time: _____

Workout 57:
3 Rounds for Time:

30 Decline Push Ups
30 Bench Dips
30 Side Small Forward Arm Circles
30 Side Small Backward Arm Circles
30 Air Overhead Press
30 V-Ups
30 Mountain Climbers
Time: _____

Workout 58:
For Time:

.5 Mile Run
50 Flutter Kicks
.5 Mile Run
50 Side-to-Side Hops (Feet Together)
.5 Mile Run
50 Standing Knee to Elbow
50 High Knees
Time: _____

Workout 59:
For Time:

100 Long Jump with Backward Jog to Start Point
100 Meter Sprint
100 Crunches
100 Russian Twists
100 Scissor Kicks
Time: _____

Workout 60:
3 Rounds for Time:

30 Wall Walks
30 Flutter Kicks
30 Push Ups
30 Laying Knee to Chest
30 Russian Twists
30 Incline Push Ups
Time: _____

Workout 61:
3 Rounds for Time:

20 Air Squats 1 and ¼
50 Standing Calf Raises 1 and ¼
20 Jumping Lunges
50 Tuck Jumps
20 Plank Crunches
50 Mountain Climbers
Time: _____

Workout 62:
3 Rounds for Time:

20 Mountain Climbers
20 Meter Bear Crawl
20 Flutter Kicks
20 V-Ups
20 Second Star Plank
20 Bench Dips
Time: _____

Workout 63:
3 Rounds for Time:

20 Incline Push Ups
20 Bench Dips
50 Jumping Jacks
20 Dive Bomber Push Ups
50 High Knees
20 Diamond Push Ups
Time: _____

Workout 64:
10 Rounds for Time:

10 Jump Squats
10 Crunches
100 Meter Sprint
10 Walking Lunges
10 Bunny Hops
Time: _____

Workout 65:
3 Rounds for Time:

25 Standing Knees-to-Elbow Cross
25 Side Small Forward Arm Circles
25 Side Small Backwards Arm Circles
25 8 Count Push Ups
25 Meter Supine Crab Walk
25 V-Ups
Time: _____

Workout 66:
3 Rounds for Time:

25 Air Squats to Calf Raise
50 Jumping Jacks
25 Speed Skaters
50 Standing Straight Leg Toe Touch
25 Bunny Hops
50 High Knees
Time: _____

Workout 67:
30-15-30

Standing Overhead Air Press
Good Mornings (Hip Hinge)
Reverse Crunches
Bench Dips
Incline Push Ups
Jumping Jacks
Time: _____

<u>Workout 68:</u>
30-20-10

1 and ¼ Air Squats
Bunny Hops
Jumping Jacks
Split Squats
Donkey Kicks
Dirty Dogs
Laying Side Leg Raises (Per Side)
Time: _____

<u>Workout 69:</u>
For Time:

100 Jumping Jacks
100 Bicycle Crunches
100 Mountain Climbers
100 Flutter Kicks
100 High Knees
Time: _____

<u>Workout 70:</u>
For Time:

100 Push Ups
100 Side Small Forward Arm Circles
100 Side Small Backwards Arm Circles
100 Mountain Climbers
100 Jumping Jacks
100 Russian Twists
Time: _____

Workout 71:
5 Rounds for Time:

10 Jumping Lunges
10 Long Jumps with Backward Jog to Start
10 Jump Squats
10 Burpees without Push Ups
Time: _____

Workout 72:
For Time:

10 Burpees
100 Scissor Kicks
Run 1.5 Miles
100 Standing Knee to Elbow Crunches
Time: _____

Workout 73:
2 Rounds for Time:

50 Standing Twists
50 Crunches
50 Flutter Kicks
50 Jumping Jacks
50 Mountain Climbers
50 High Knees
Time: _____

Workout 74:
30-20-20

Donkey Kicks
Dirty Dogs
Laying Side Leg Raise (Per Side)
Chair/Bench Step Ups
Bunny Hops
Jumping Jacks
Flutter Kicks
Time: _____

Workout 75:
4 Rounds for Time:

30 Second Wall Sit
15 1 and ¼ Air Squats
30 Speed Skaters
15 Lunges at 45 Degree (Per Side)
30 V-Ups
15 Plank Rolls (1 = Left Side to-Regular Plank-to-Right)
Time: _____

Workout 76:
3 Rounds for Time:

45 Second Wall Sit
45 Second Plank
45 Second Left Side Plank
45 Second Right Side Plank
45 Plank Crunches
Time: _____

<u>Workout 77</u>:
3 Rounds for Time:

20 High Knees
20 Burpees
20 Dive Bomber Push Ups
20 Bench Dips
20 Incline Push Ups
20 V-Ups
Time: _____

<u>Workout 78</u>:
3 Rounds for Time:

20 Squats
20 Meters of High Skipping Running Drill
20 Lunges
100 Meter Sprint
20 Burpees
Time: _____

<u>Workout 79</u>:
For Time:

100 Jumping Jacks
100 Bunny Hops
100 High Knees
100 Russian Twists
100 Chair Squats
Time: _____

Workout 80:
3 Rounds for Time:

50 Jumping Air Squats
25 Plank Crunches
50 Side Lunges (25 Each Side)
25 Calf Raises 1 and ¼
50 Side-to-Side Hops (Feet Together)
Time: _____

Workout 81:
3 Rounds for Time:

50 Side Small Arm Circles Backward
25 Bicycle Crunches
50 Mountain Climbers
25 Overhead Air Press
50 Side Small Arm Circles Forward
25 V-Ups
Time: _____

Workout 82:
For Time:

50 Mountain Climbers
50 Jumping Jacks
50 Speed Skaters
50 High Knees
50 Standing Knee to Elbow Crunch
Time: _____

Workout 83:
3 Rounds for Time:

25 Squat Jumps
50 Reverse Crunches
25 Dirty Dogs (Per Side)
50 Standing Calf Raise 1 and ¼
25 Donkey Kicks (Per Side)
50 Russian Twists
Time: _____

Workout 84:
3 Rounds for Time:

20 Hand Walkouts (Plank Walkout)
20 Meter Supine Crab Walk
20 Incline Push Ups
20 Bench Dips
20 Decline Push Ups
20 Meter Bear Crawl
Time: _____

Workout 85:
5 Rounds for Time:

25 Squat Jumps (Jump Squats)
25 Meters Sprint
25 High Knees
30 Jumping Lunges
30 Standing Knee to Elbow Crunches
Time: _____

Workout 86:
1-10 Pyramid of Push Ups with 10 Standing Knee to Elbow & 10 OH Presses After Each Set of Push Ups

After each Push Up set:
10 Standing Knee to Elbow
10 Overhead Air Press

Example of Workout:
1 Push Up
10 Standing Knee to Elbow
10 Overhead Air Press

2 Push Ups
10 Standing Knee to Elbow
10 Overhead Air Press

3 Push Ups
10 Standing Knee to Elbow
10 Overhead Air Press

Continue until reach 10 Push Ups
Time: _____

Workout 87:
5 Rounds for Time:

20 Jump Squats
20 Split Squats (10 each Leg)
50 Bicycle Crunches
Time: _____

Workout 88:
3 Rounds for Time:

30 Bench Dips
30 Meter Bear Crawl
30 Side Forward Small Arm Circles
30 Side Backward Arm Circles
30 Overhead Air Press
30 Push Ups
30 Standing Knee to Elbow
Time: _____

Workout 89:
5 Rounds for Time:

20 Jump Squats
20 Meter Sprint (Hill if available)
20 Burpees
20 Standing Knee to Elbow
20 Lunges (10 Each Leg)
Time: _____

Workout 90:
3 Rounds for Time:

20 Incline Push Ups
20 Bicycle Crunches
20 Mountain Climbers
20 Plank Crunches
20 Russian Twists
Time: _____

Workout 91:
20-15-10

Decline Push Ups
V-Ups
Bench Dips
Burpees without Push Up
Alternating Toe Taps
Time: _____

Workout 92:
3 Rounds for Time:

20 Meter Bear Crawl
50 Mountain Climbers
20 Meter Supine Crab Walk
50 High Knees
20 Jumping Jacks
50 Side to Side Hop (Feet Together)
Time: _____

Workout 93:
3 Rounds for Time:

50 Incline Push Ups
50 Flutter Kicks
50 Bench Dips
50 Jumping Leg Scissors
50 Mountain Climbers
50 Russian Twists
Time: _____

Workout 94:
3 Rounds for Time:

50 Bench/Chair Step Ups (25 Each Leg)
30 Jump Squats
50 Bunny Hops
30 Jumping Lunges
50 Donkey Kicks (25 Each Leg)
30 Standing Knee to Elbow
Time: _____

Workout 95:
3 Rounds for Time:

25 Push Ups
25 V-Ups
25 Incline Push Ups
25 Plank Crunches
25 Close Grip Push Ups
25 V-Ups
Time: _____

Workout 96:
3 Rounds for Time:

25 Tuck Jumps
30 Jumping Lunges
35 Standing Calf Raise 1 and ¼
40 Side to Side Hops (Feet Together)
45 Laying Pulse Up
50 Mountain Climbers
Time: _____

Workout 97:
For Time:

.5 Miles
50 Jumping Jacks
.5 Miles
50 Flutter Kicks
Time: _____

Workout 98:
3 Rounds for Time:

30 Side Large Forward Arm Circles
30 Push Ups
30 V-Ups
30 Chair Handstand Push Ups
30 Bench Dips
30 Bicycle Crunches
30 Side Large Backward Arm Circles
30 Overhead Air Press
Time: _____

Workout 99:
3 Rounds for Time:

50 Jumping Jacks
50 ¼ Air Squats
500 Meters Jog/Run
50 Bunny Hops
50 Standing Knee to Elbow Crunch
50 High Knees
Time: _____

<u>Workout 100:</u>
30-20-10

Jump Squats
Sit Ups
Walking Lunges
Chair Step Ups
Straight Leg Toe Touches
Laying Scissor Kicks
Time: _____

<u>Workout 101:</u>
For Time:

50 High Knees
50 Side Small Forward Arm Circles
50 Side Small Backward Arm Circles
50 Overhead Air Press
50 Mountain Climbers
50 Incline Push Ups
Time: _____

<u>Workout 102:</u>
3 Rounds for Time:

20 Air Squats 1 and ¼
20 Burpees without Push Ups
20 Lunges
20 Bunny Hops
20 Standing Knee to Elbow Crunch
20 Speed Skaters
Time: _____

Workout 103:
3 Rounds for Time:

25 Bench Dips
25 Side Small Forward Arm Circles
25 Side Small Backwards Arm Circles
25 Front Arm Circles Both Ways
25 Incline Push Ups
25 Crunches
25 Standing Knee to Elbow
Time: _____

Workout 104:
3 Rounds for Time:

25 Wall Walks
25 Bicycle Crunches
25 Diamond Push Ups
25 Toe Taps (Per Foot)
Dolphin Kicks
25 Mountain Climbers
25 Kneeling Back Extension
Time: _____

Workout 105:
5 Rounds for Time:

10 Tuck Jumps
100 Meter Sprint
100-Meter Run Alternating High Skip Drill
10 Burpees
Time: _____

Workout 106:
3 Rounds for Time:

50 Standing Scissor Jumps
50 Bicycle Crunches
50 Flutter Kicks
50 Jumping Jacks
50 Laying Scissor Kicks
50 Standing Knee to Elbow Crunch
50 Mountain Climbers
Time: _____

Workout 107:
10 Rounds for Time:

10 8-Count Push Ups
50 Meter Run
10 Reverse Crunches
10 Russian Twists
Time: _____

Workout 108:
30-20-10

1 and ¼ Air Squats
Standing Straight Leg Toe Touch
Lunges
1 and ¼ Standing Calf Raise
High Knees
Speed Skaters
Time: _____

Workout 109:
For Time:

20 Meter Straight Leg Bound Drill
2 Mile Run
20 Standing Knee to Elbow
Time: _____

Workout 110:
2 Rounds for Time:

50 Bicycle Crunches
50 Sit Ups
10 Long Jump with Backward Jog to Start Point
1-Mile Jog
50 Alternating Toe Taps
50 Mountain Climbers
Time: _____

Workout 111:
3 Rounds for Time:

20 Side-to-Side Hop (Feet Together)
20 High Knees
20 V-Ups
20 Ab Scissors
20 Plank Crunches
20 Burpees
Time: _____

Workout 112:
3 Rounds for Time:

20 Jumping Squats
20 Jumping Lunges
20 45-Degree Forward Lunge (Per Side)
50 Jumping Jacks
50 Second Wall Sit
50 V-Ups
Time: _____

Workout 113:
3 Rounds for Time:

20 Laying Leg Raises (90 Degree)
20 Chair Handstand Push Ups
20 Bicycle Crunches
20 Decline Push Ups
40 Jumping Jacks
60 Seconds of Plank Rolls (Left, Reg., Right)
Time: _____

Workout 114:
3 Rounds for Time:

20 Tuck Jumps
20 Jumping Lunges
20 Bunny Hops
20 Standing Knees-to-Elbow Crossover
20 Speed Skaters
20 High Knees
Time: _____

Workout 115:
3 Rounds for Time:

20 Reverse Crunches
20 Russian Twists
20 ¼ Crunches
20 Standing Knee to Elbows
20 Mountain Climbers
20 Side to Side Hop (Feet Together)
Time: _____

Workout 116:
3 Rounds for Time:

20 Incline Push Ups
50 Jumping Jacks
20 Decline Push Ups
50 Jumping Jacks
20 Push Ups
50 Jumping Jacks
Time: _____

Workout 117:
3 Rounds for Time:

60 Seconds of Reg. Plank
30 Mountain Climbers
60 Seconds of Left/Right Side Plank (30 each)
30 Jumping Jacks
60 Alternating Toe Taps
Time: _____

Workout 118:
30-20-30

High Knees
Speed Skaters
Mountain Climbers
Ab Wipers
Plank Crunches
Bunny Hops
Side-to-Side Hop (Feet Together)
Time: _____

Workout 119:
5 Rounds for Time:

15 Meter Bear Crawl
30 Mountain Climbers
15 8-Count Push Ups
30 Jumping Jacks
15 Supine Crab Walk
Time: _____

Workout 120:
3 Rounds for Time:

10 Burpees
20 Jumping Squats
30 Jumping Lunges
40 Standing Calf Raise 1 and ¼
50 High Knees
50 Speed Skaters
Time: _____

Workout 121:
3 Rounds for Time:

30 Donkey Kicks
30 Standing Straight Leg Toe Touches
30 Standing Knee to Elbow
30 Dirty Dogs
30 Laying Side Leg Raise (Per Leg)
Time: _____

Workout 122:
3 Rounds for Time:

10 Burpees with Push Up
50 Standing Scissor Kick Jumps
500 Meter Run
50 Mountain Climbers
10 Meter Backward Sprint
Time: _____

Workout 123:
3 Rounds for Time:

50 Half Wiper Abs
50 Reverse Crunches
50 Push Ups
50 Second Star Plank Hold
50 Second Bridge Plank Hold
50 Alternating Toe Taps
50 High Knees
Time: _____

Workout 124:
3 Rounds for Time:

20 Russian Twists
10 Burpees without Push Ups
10 8-Count Push Ups
20 Bench Dips
10 V-Ups
10 Meter Supine Crab Walk
20 Reverse Flutter Kicks
Time: _____

Workout 125:
10 Rounds for Time:

10 Tuck Jumps
20 Meter Sprint
30 Standing Calf Raise 1 and ¼
40 Mountain Climbers
50 Alternating Toe Taps
Time: _____

Workout 126:
For Time:

1 Mile Run
100 Push Ups
100 Crunches
100 Sitting Punches (½ up on Sit Up)
100 Standing Scissor Kick Jumps
Time: _____

Workout 127:
3 Rounds for Time:

20 Donkey Kicks (Per Leg)
20 Dirty Dogs (Per Leg)
20 Air Squats 1 and ¼
20 Speed Skaters
20 Standing Straight Leg Touch
Time: _____

Workout 128:
3 Rounds for Time:

30 Good Mornings (Hip Hinge)
10 Plank Walkouts
30 Push Ups
10 Reverse Snow Angel
30 Seconds of Wall Walks
10 Plank Crunches
30 Flutter Kicks
Time: _____

Workout 129:
30-20-15

Jumping Squats
High Knees
Jumping Jacks
Bunny Hops
Split Squats
Leg Lifts
Time: _____

Workout 130:
5 Rounds for Time:

30 Standing Scissor Kick Jumps
30 Meter Sprint
30 Meter Backward Sprint
30 Meter Crossover Drill Left
30 Meter Crossover Drill Right
30 High Knees
Time: _____

Workout 131:
3 Rounds for Time:

20 Meter Bear Crawl
20 Meter Crab Walk
20 Standing Elbow to Knee Crunch
20 Plank Crunches (10 Per Side)
20 Plank Walkouts (Hand Walkout)
20 Standing Core Twists
Time: _____

Workout 132:
30-20-30

Reverse Flutter Kicks
Incline Close Grip Push Ups
Good Mornings (Hip Hinge)
Vertical Leg Crunches
Bicycle Crunches
Alternating Ankle Touch
Time: _____

Workout 133:
3 Rounds for Time:

20 Air Squats 1 and ¼
20 Jumping Lunges
20 Side to Side Hops (Feet Together)
20 Step Ups
20 Speed Skaters
20 Jumping Jacks
20 V-Ups
Time: _____

Workout 134:
9 Minutes or 3 Rounds:

60 Seconds Plank
30 Seconds Left Plank (30 Seconds Right)
30 Seconds Bridge Pose
30 Seconds of Star Plank
-No Time-

Workout 135:
3 Rounds for Time:

25 Bench Dips
25 Flutter Kicks
25 Small Arm Circles Forward
25 Small Arm Circles Backward
25 Overhead Air Press
25 Decline Push Ups
25 Reverse Crunches
Time: _____

Workout 136:
5 Rounds for Time:

5 Burpees
5 Dive Bomber Push Ups
10 Standing Elbow to Knee
10 Long Jump with Backward Jog to Start Point
20 Jumping Jacks
20 High Knees
Time: _____

Workout 137:
3 Rounds for Time:

20 Split Squats
20 Standing Straight Leg Toe Touches
20 Donkey Kicks
20 Left and Right-Side Laying Leg Lifts
20 Dirty Dogs
20 Bunny Hops
20 Jumping Jacks
Time: _____

Workout 138:
3 Rounds for Time:

20 Crunches
20 Reverse Crunches
20 Flutter Kicks
20 Russian Twists
20 Ab Wipers
Time: _____

Workout 139:
5 Rounds for Time:

20 Standing Elbow to Knee Crunch
20 Jumping Jacks
20 Mountain Climbers
20 V-Ups
20 High Knees
20 Side to Side Hops (Feet Together)
Time: _____

Workout 140:
5 Rounds for Time:

20 Second Star Plank
20 Hand Walkouts (Plank Walkouts)
20 Push Ups
20 Second L-Sit
20 Bicycle Crunches
20 Bench Dips
Time: _____

Workout 141:
30-20-10

Jump Squats
Jumping Lunges
Long Jump with Backward Jog to Start Point
Bunny Hops
Donkey Kicks
Laying Leg Lifts (Per Side)
Time: _____

Workout 142:
3 Rounds for Time:

100 Meter Sprint
20 Plank Crunches
100 Jumping Jacks
20 Russian Twists
100 High Knees
Time: _____

Workout 143:
3 Rounds for Time:

10 Burpees with Push Ups
30 Second Plank
30 Second Left/Right Plank (15 Per Side)
30 Second Bridge Pose
30 Mountain Climbers
30 Speed Skaters
1 Minute of Shadow Boxing (Work Angles/Light Feet)
Time: _____

Workout 144:
20-15-10

Dolphin Kicks
8 Count Push Ups
3 Count Good Mornings
4 Count Jumping Jacks
Forward/Backward Large Arm Circles (Reps Per)
Reverse Crunches
Time: _____

Workout 145:
5 Rounds for Time:

20 Split Squats
20 Standing Straight Leg Toe Touch
20 Step Ups
20 Standing 1 and ¼ Calf Raises
20 Standing Elbow to Knee Crunch
20 Crunches
Time: _____

Workout 146:
5 Rounds for Time:

20 High Knees
20 Meter Crossover Running Drill (L&R Side)
20 Meters of Straight Leg Bound Drill
20 Meter Sprint
20 Meter Backward Jog/Sprint
20 Plank Crunches
Time: _____

Workout 147:
3 Rounds for Time:

20 Incline Push Ups
20 Meter Bear Crawl
20 Meter Supine Crab Walk
20 Standing Overhead Air Press
20 Air Swimmers (On Stomach)
20 Ab Wipers
Time: _____

Workout 148:
3 Rounds for Time:

20 Incline Push Ups
20 Bench Dips
20 Decline Push Ups
20 Second Star Plank
20 Second L-Sit
20 Wall Walks or HSPU
Time: _____

Workout 149:
3 Rounds for Time:

20 Speed Skaters
20 Straight Leg High Kicks (Per Leg)
20 Dirty Dogs (Per Leg)
20 Donkey Kicks (Per Leg)
20 Sitting Punches (Abs)
20 Straight Leg Toe Touches
Time: _____

Workout 150:
For Time:

100 Push Ups
100 Sit Ups
100 Russian Twists
100 Jumping Jacks
100 High Knees
100 Standing Elbow to Knee Crunch
Time: _____

CPSIA information can be obtained
at www.ICGtesting.com
Printed in the USA
BVHW031942240320
575859BV00001B/53